C.P.R.
Choice Processing and Resolution

C.P.R.
Choice Processing and Resolution

Facing Grief After Abortion Without Fear

TRUDY JOHNSON M.A., L.M.F.T.

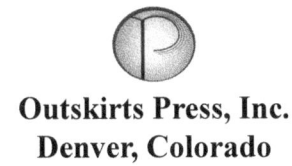

Outskirts Press, Inc.
Denver, Colorado

Jesse Lynn, the missing piece to my heart

To the disenfranchised voices of "vpt"

C.P.R.
Choice Processing and Resolution
All Rights Reserved.
Copyright © 2010 Trudy M. Johnson
V3.0 R4

Cover Photo © 2009 JupiterImages Corporation. All rights reserved - used with permission.

Outskirts Press, Inc.
http://www.outskirtspress.com

ISBN: 978-1-4327-4329-1

Library of Congress Control Number: 2009930193

Outskirts Press and the "OP" logo are trademarks belonging to Outskirts Press, Inc.

PRINTED IN THE UNITED STATES OF AMERICA

Acknowledgements

To my faithful friend and editor, Barb

To the constant inspirations of my life,
my two sons, Jobie and Jerret

To my soul mate and encourager, my husband, Lonney

THE HARDEST PART OF THE JOURNEY OF 1,000 MILES
IS THE FIRST BRAVE STEP.

What Others Are Saying:

"Trudy helped me through a difficult time in my life. The compassion she has for the "vpt" woman is evident. This resource has calmed the storm in my soul. I am so grateful she had the courage to broach this subject."

"Jill" "vpt" woman, Colorado

"Finally! I am so grateful for "CPR." It is so nice to know that I am not crazy! It was hard to look at my "vpt" but once I did with the help of this book, I am in a whole new place with my life."

Liz "vpt" woman, California

"This is the book I wish I would have found ten years ago. Finally! I've found a common sense way to process my past abortion. This resource was very helpful for me to get to the bottomline and work through to a better place with my "vpt.""

Mary "vpt" woman, Texas

"CPR" is a wonderful combination of compassion and professionalism that speaks to the "vpt" woman in no other way. I am so grateful for this resource that I will be giving out to my future clients."

Terrie Lenzini, LPC, Colorado

"I have one girl I'm working with who stopped counting at five "vpt" decisions. She is having a hard time processing anything. Wow, I loaned her the "CPR" book. I believe she is starting to feel again. Thank you!

Robin P., RN, Indiana
(STARS Leader)

"Trudy, Bravo! I've long known about the need for grieving voluntary pregnancy termination. I've also written about this, but you've taken the subject to a whole new level. I'll be featuring C.P.R.~ Choice Processing and Resolution as a resource in my new revised book, Women's Bodies, Women's Wisdom."

Dr. Christiane Northrup, M.D. F.A.C.O.G.

Table of Contents

Notes to the Reader

For Women, Men, Parents and Friends

If you've picked up this book, it's either because you, your partner, your wife, your daughter, your sibling, your friend, or someone else close to you have a choice decision in their past they need to resolve because they are experiencing grief and sadness. Your motivation may be out of curiosity to learn what others may have experienced because of a past choice decision. You may be seeking information on how to help someone near and dear to you who is suffering depression because of a voluntary pregnancy termination. You may have helped someone make the decision. You may have kept quiet and not entered into the choice- making process at all. Maybe you, like so many others need your own personal resolution to this issue. Even though this writing speaks directly to the woman who made the choice, this book also provides helpful information for those standing on the sidelines as well.

Why is this book different?

This is the only book available in the history of choice that addresses *only* the grief component of choice decisions. It is a non-judgmental presentation for all faiths and cultures. *C.P.R.* ~ *Choice Processing and Resolution* is literally a "first aid kit" that helps process and resolve your voluntary pregnancy termination in a compassionate, safe atmosphere. Tears are allowed. Judgment and condemnation are *not*.

Do You Need to Talk?

Evidence shows that only about one in ten women have ever shared their abortion secret with another person. *No one* talks about their deep dark secret because of fear of receiving condemnation or invalidation.

Trudy offers her time to you as a safe place to share your voluntary pregnancy termination story and receive help from a compassionate, professional source.

You may go to the Web site, www.missingpieces.org and choose eTherapi or Skype in the navigation bar to request your *hippa-compliant* video call appointment with Trudy.

Calls from women, men, family members, friends and professional therapists needing guidance with clients are welcomed. All credit cards accepted for appointments.

YOU NEVER HAVE TO FEEL ALONE IN THIS JOURNEY

JOIN OUR COMMUNITY

FACEBOOK:

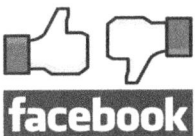

C.P.R.~Choice Processing and Resolution has a Facebook page at this address: https://www.facebook.com/dealingwithgriefafterabortion

Receive encouragement or private message Trudy from this page.

READ TRUDY'S BLOG AND ARTICLES:
Trudy Johnson is the "expert on grief after abortion" on the Your Tango.com Web site.

Read Trudy's blog and articles on the Your Tango.com Web site here: http://www.yourtango.com/experts/trudyjohnson

You can also send Trudy a private message from her Your Tango. com page.

EMAIL TRUDY:
You may send Trudy a confidential note or your personal story to missingpiecesorg@gmail.com

No abusive or political statements please

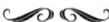

Every choice, every decision has its own unique set of circumstances. The life situations we were in were so varied. But our commonality is the same.

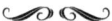

For so many women, it is hard for them to connect themselves to the "A-word" for fear of condemnation or because of shame.

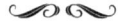

Just as a voluntary pregnancy termination shouldn't be available only from a backroom entrance, *processing and resolving that choice* shouldn't have to be done in secret for fear of disclosure not being a safe place or of minimizing, condemnation or shaming confrontation.

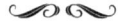

1

An Introduction to C.P.R.

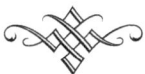

It is no accident you are reading this book. You may have taken many roads in your life. Now you're at an intersection. This book brings you answers to help you care for a deep place in your heart that might be painful and confusing for you. Pain is a universal language that needs no interpreter. It doesn't matter your race, your religion, or your geographic location, pain is now the common bond you hold with other women who feel a need to re-visit a time and place from their past.

There is one thing you need to know: *"You are not alone."* There are many, many others who relate to your heart's cry. My journey started where you are right now. Others' journeys are starting this same day in the same way your journey is beginning this very moment. We are women who are "keepers of the secret" and we all need a safe place to cry. You need to know you are not alone. I myself have "been there" just as countless other women all across the world.

Voluntary pregnancy termination is not anything we set out to do as a "goal" *per se*. It was never any of our basic desires to have to *choose*. Just like we were all on different roads and now we are here at this intersection, so are the choices we've made. Every choice, every decision has its own unique set of circumstances. The life situations we were in were so varied. But our commonality is the same.

There were other choices we *could* have made. Single-parenting, "having to get married," adoption or in the case of a tough medical outcome…none of the options available provided perfect answers. For many of us perfection was demanded from us, either by ourselves or by others. Choices, decisions are hard. There is never any easy answer.

Every single one of the roads we *could* have chosen involve loss and grief. The only difference in "our choice" and the other choices we could/would/should have made is that the "other choices" have external results. All of the other choices available to us had elements of connection to them. Single-parenting, marriage, adoption…there is some component of human attachment and/or bonding to them. In voluntary termination, we take the solitary road.

We take the road alone and for most of us we are unable to talk to anyone about it. The world in general, others, and even we "assume" we are fine. And well we may be. In voluntary termination, there is no evidence of a baby…there is no "missing person" in our lives and the father may already be out of the picture. We get up and go on with our lives… without relationship. We are in one sense relieved to "get on with the business of living" and we file our decision away as anything from "barely a blip on the radar screen," to "I'm so sad I could die."

As time passes and our lives return to balance---it may be a day, weeks, months or even several years---an unusual thing starts happening. A deep sense of loss may begin to surface. The craziest thing might "trigger us." For me, it was a cold March day. I was in the super market shopping, rounded the corner and ran into another shopper with a beautiful little girl seated in her cart. Her curls looked like angel curls and her eyes were the bluest I've ever seen. Suddenly a sense of sadness overcame me that I was unable to shake off.

I ended up leaving the store, running out to my car and crying. It wouldn't be until a few years later that I realized this incident coincided with the anniversary of the voluntary termination of my pregnancy. That too happened to be a "cold March day."

I've talked with many other ladies, including many clients who detail to me similar experiences. One person was walking through the baby department in a big clothing store. The other lady drove by a playground and saw the children playing on the swings.

This sense of loss is very normal and it may take years before experiencing it. After the supermarket incident I began to think about the termination, but of course did not dialogue with *anyone*. After all, exactly *who in the* world could I talk with about my feelings? I eventually came to the dead end conclusion that there was no way I had a "right to grieve" a loss that I was responsible for. What I'd done was legal. I must be crazy to be feeling so sad.

So I walked the road alone realizing that voluntary pregnancy termination is a choice I made on my own. I concluded therefore that processing any overflow emotional responses regarding the termination of the pregnancy were also up to me, just as much of the choice decision had been.

Feeling the responsibility of the choice and feeling like there is no allowance for grieving a loss one has *chosen* are a few of the various reasons women don't talk about their voluntary termination of pregnancy. For the most part it is for fear of condemnation, discounting and minimizing our situation. We even have the conversation with *ourselves*. "I chose this as a solution to my crisis, so why should I feel bad, why should I feel sad, why should I feel anything at all?" Unfortunately, there are no answers and no one to voice any sort of hopeful message about the turmoil going on in the inside.

I myself found nowhere to run when I began feeling confusion and pain because of the loss I experienced years ago. It is for this reason I feel compelled to send down a lifeline to my sisters of choice. I hope this book will bring some answers for your questions and give you a helpful plan for resolution to the voluntary termination of your pregnancy.

Why Do I Refer to the "A-word" as "vpt?"

There are a few parameters for processing and resolving your pregnancy termination through the use of this book. First and most important is that you understand that you are not alone. I know I keep saying these words, but just realize that the "A" club we belong to is much greater than one might think. You may be alone reading this book, but you are not alone with your questions, confusion and/or pain.

Secondly, I am *choosing* not to use the "A-word" in this book. The "A-word" has the potential of adding to the confusion as you process and reconcile your choice. I've crafted the term "Voluntary Pregnancy Termination" or the acronym "vpt" as a way to refer to the "procedure." This gets the terminology out of the realm of any preconceived ideas you might have about your "vpt" resolution. The "A-word" incites many heated discussions.

It is much more important for you to be able to face your choice and process the grief and reach resolution than for you to dialogue political and religious arguments in your head. For so many women I've worked with, it is hard for them to connect themselves with the

AN INTRODUCTION TO C.P.R.

"A-word." They are at a different place in life and they are unable to look at themselves in the present as "that person." There can be so much shame and condemnation involved. Again, we walk the solitary road when it comes to talking about our choices.

I will always remember a 62 year-old client who was coming to me for grief resolution. She disclosed that on all the medical forms she'd filled out through the years, she had never written the "A" word on her intake information. She could not make the connection from her head to writing the word on the paper.

"Vpt" was our personal decision; it is the common bond that unites us. We are the ones who know what "vpt" is about. "Vpt" is my personal journey and my own unique experience that has nothing to do with political discussion. There is no doubt in my mind that many news commentators don't understand what "vpt" has meant to me on a personal heart level. Most professional counselors don't understand, the majority of pastors don't understand, many of my friends don't understand and I would say *all* of my family members don't understand. You the reader, however, understand what I am saying. I the writer understand your journey, your heart. We have commonalities that those who speak like experts, yet who couldn't possibly understand, don't. So "vpt" is what I will refer to from here on out. I hope this change in label will help you move out of that vague place of denial. You now have permission to process your loss. You are free to look at the grief you might be experiencing over your "vpt."

Just as a voluntary pregnancy termination shouldn't be available only from a backroom entrance, *processing and resolving* our choice shouldn't have to be done in secret for fear of disclosure. My personal journey of resolution involved several years. I was confused and in pain but only received answers from random sources. We shouldn't have to risk rejection, condemnation, misunderstanding or disapproval just because we are searching for resolution. Also, I believe that keeping all concepts of "vpt" in the political realm stops us from allowing processing when the time comes for that.

Those who've chosen "vpt" shouldn't have to assume that if we even ask questions we are putting choice in jeopardy of losing its legal status.

This mind-set is an archaic one. Imagine if a person suffering from alcoholism were afraid to get help because it might cause the nation to go back into the era of prohibition. It should not only be "OK" to get help to process "vpt" - it should be absolutely acceptable in the eyes of our culture.

C.P.R. ~ Choice Processing and Resolution is a way for those struggling with their grief to finally "have permission" to "go there" with their emotions and their questions. Finally, those who've chosen all over the world can grieve, process and reconcile the loss incurred through "vpt." Again, no more hiding about the grief that accompanies a voluntary termination of pregnancy!

You will read my story in the next chapter, but for right now, just know that when it came my time to grieve there was no one available to help me. I went to a professional counselor and two pastors and only walked away with more sadness and confusion. It is important for you to know that *"you are not alone"* and others have been in the exact same place you are right now. I was also one of those women.

Understanding the Importance of Safety

I hope you will let this time of intersecting roads be a place of safety and comfort. It is very likely that only a few people, if *anyone*, know about your experience with "vpt." Processing and reconciling your choice, your secret, might bring up some emotion you've pushed down for years. You may be bringing up and out some feelings you have *never* allowed yourself to have. For this reason, you need to be very safe physically, emotionally, mentally and spiritually while you read this book.

As a licensed professional therapist, I have become increasingly aware that our women are suffering greatly from lack of care, comfort and nurturing. Many women did not get this from their mothers, much less their fathers. Somewhere in their quest to "have it all" women have lost the fine art of comforting themselves. In her book, *A Gift from the Sea,* Anne Morrow Lindbergh makes the very wise comment, "What a circus act we women perform everyday of our lives. This is not the life of simplicity, but the life of multiplicity that the wise men warn us of. It leads not to unification but to fragmentation. It does not bring grace; it destroys the soul." Women run on empty fumes in their tank. As a result, they get less and less efficient, less and less at peace with their souls.

While you are reading this book, just know that now is your time to be safe. You are reading words penned by a writer who has compassion for you. This book is a safe place to read about and process your secret. So let this journey be one of safety and comfort as you walk with others who are in the exact same life situation as you.

I would suggest reading this book in the privacy of your own home. Reading while you are on a plane or at work would not be the ideal setting for delving into your resolution process. Creating safety is something you can do on your own. I actually have what I call a "safe place" in my home.

My hope is that you might be able to create such a place in yours. Actually, all the homes I've lived in over the past couple of decades have had a "safe place." Will you think me strange if I admit to you that at one point I lived in an apartment that had a *huge* bathroom and I was able to make this my "safe place"? I put a wonderful pillow on the floor and beside me was a small stereo that provided soothing music when I needed it. Anytime I wanted to get away I could always go into my bathroom and close the door.

Presently, my "safe place" is much more practical, but still very simple. It's a small sofa in my office with a soft lamp sitting on a table with probably anywhere from six to twenty books lying nearby. The most important component of my safe place is "my blankee." Again, I am being very vulnerable here…me a grown woman admitting that I have a "blankee." It is amazing the softness of baby blankets these days. I have an actual real baby blanket that I can sit and cover myself with. The blanket was expensive for a baby's blanket…around $20.00…but all in all one of the best investments I've ever made. It is soft like a cloud and just plain *exudes* safety and non-judgment. I add to this a nice cup of French vanilla coffee and I have my safe haven, an instant vacation from the worries and insanity of the world. And so it is that I would suggest you also be creative in finding your own little slot, a corner that you can call your own as you walk this journey. Again, you may have to be very creative in making your nest, but if I can turn a bathroom into a sanctuary, I know you can also find a place where you can pull away from the distractions around you to start your own choice resolution.

This book is in your hands for a reason. It is "your time" to courageously face what your soul already knows. You made a choice in a circumstance that demanded you make it. Choosing means you took one road and left another road behind. You have permission, now is the time!

Who Are We?

I keep mentioning the fact that you are not alone. I think it important to interject information about the demographics of the woman of choice in our nation. Women who've voluntarily terminated pregnancies are everywhere! We consist of every ethnicity, every religion, every economic class. We are career women, we are moms, we are grandmothers, we are aunts, we are sisters. We could be your next door neighbor or even your pastor's wife.

Planned Parenthood does an excellent job of keeping track of how many procedures are performed throughout the years. You can go to the statistical gathering arm of their organization called the Alan Guttmacher Institute (www.agi-org) to find any mathematical information you would like. For simplicity sake, though, let me help you understand the facts and figures of voluntary pregnancy termination.

For the past years since the legalization of choice in 1973, there has been an *average* of 1.2-1.5 million "vpt" decisions every year. In a world where trillion is a household word, I think a word picture of actual warm bodies would be helpful. Let's look at pro-football to give you an idea of just how many of us have made choice decisions. At the writing of this book there are ten National League Football teams and ten American League Football teams. Each team's stadium holds anywhere from 50,000 to 100,000 plus fans. If we (for sake of this word picture) say the average stadium holds 60,000 fans, then you can look at the number of "vpt" choices in our nation each year *as every single football league's stadium full of people at the same time.* That would be all 20 stadiums filled to the brim with women! Now I can't quite imagine the amount of words or the number of potty breaks you would count in a scene like this, but I hope you get the picture. Women who've made a decision to voluntarily terminate a pregnancy are the largest demographic in our nation. As you can see, *you are not alone!*

I made my choice decision at age twenty,
so "vpt" has been a part of my entire adult life.

I had a horrible feeling in the pit of my stomach but I felt like
this was my only way out. I didn't think about the pregnancy as a
pregnancy. Mostly, it was an inconvenient situation, a crisis that I
really needed out of my way as soon as possible.

I didn't feel like I had the right to grieve my loss --there was no
external evidence of a baby… and I didn't feel like I should be
allowed permission to grieve over a loss that I had chosen.

2

"Go Home and Get Over It"

We all have our stories. This book begins with my story, but you will have your chance to tell your story. Telling the story allows us to get things up and out. Up and out releases the pain. We process. We find resolution. We reach a place of peace.

For most of us, our stories are buried as far down as possible. If you are reading this book it is my guess that you have not shared your secret with anyone, or at least with only a few people whom you consider safe. We don't talk about it out of fear of condemnation, invalidation or just plain shame. It is human nature to avoid the risk of disapproval. For this reason, we keep our secret very well protected.

As a licensed professional therapist, the oldest client I've had was a 96 year-old woman who experienced a voluntary pregnancy termination in her early 30's. She almost went to her grave with her secret. In desperation, though, she wanted someone to hear her story. I listened with compassion and understanding. I felt privileged to be a safe place for her. There is something very healing about sharing life's losses with others. Weeping with this dear soul is one of my most treasured professional memories. Such a long time to keep a secret!

C.P.R.

I made my choice at age twenty, so "vpt" has been a part of my entire adult life. I've walked the road of choice and having done so feel I have the credibility to walk along side others experiencing pain or confusion from their "vpt" loss.

I was 20 years old, a sophomore in college when I found myself in an unplanned pregnancy. I was the only one in my family who'd ever gone to college. I had a full ride scholarship and there was "no way" I could face my parents or even myself by changing the course of my goals. The father was in the same situation. He was the only one in his family who had been to college. He was on work study with NASA, a coveted spot to be in and too valuable to give up for any reason. This was "his shot" at life. Please know that the object of this writing is not to bash my boyfriend and former husband in this "vpt" decision. Ultimately, I accept full responsibility for the "vpt" choice.

While recounting all the details is helpful in resolution, I remember very little about the days prior to the "vpt." I will tell you what I know only because I will be asking you to do the same exercise. I remember sitting in my doctor's office feeling very alone, overwhelmed, mostly in unbelief. I felt like I was in a car that had just slammed into a brick wall. There was "no way out" of this mess. I remember envisioning my Dad and my Mom's face and how disappointed they would be. I did feel anger towards myself for being so stupid. I think the first doctor appointment could best be described as denial. I kept thinking the answer would be different than what I suspected.

When I told the father (now my ex-husband) the news he was angry. He told me there was only "one solution" to our situation. He would consider nothing else. Since I was feeling so much shame and worry about telling my parents I agreed with him. I had a horrible feeling in the pit of my stomach but I felt like this was my only way out. I didn't think about the pregnancy as a pregnancy.

Mostly, it was an inconvenient situation, a crisis that I really needed out of my way as soon as possible. I did not connect in anyway that this was a pregnancy.

I only remember two or three things about "the day." I remember it was cold and windy, a March day. And then I remember that my boyfriend said, "It's over, it's done and we will never talk about this again." And so the secret began. I did what he said. I never talked again until I was able to find a safe place to share my secret. This was over 20 years after the fact.

I do remember getting in the car and driving off. Mostly, I felt numb and did not think about this day for many, many years. Immediately, my first reaction was relief. Probably a bit like feeling you'd just been pardoned from a prison sentence.

It was about nine years later that "things" started surfacing. I am really one to believe that all things happen for a reason. My "vpt" resolution began with a book coming across my path. This is why I feel that there is a reason this book is in your hands. There are no accidents! Unfortunately, I do not remember the name, author or any details of the book. I only remember the writer detailing the events after attending her first child's funeral. *"A piece of my soul was buried with my child that day."* It was a short sentence that would forever impact my life.

I began a quest for answers to the pain I was feeling. I was in a constant dialogue with myself. My thought patterns were bouncing back and forth between, "I don't feel anything" to "I feel everything." "I shouldn't be feeling anything" to "I feel a whole bunch of everything." On and on…various different dialogues in my head with opposing patterns of consistency and sense. It was truly "crazy-making." Each day I tried to find ways to stuff the feelings. I avoided the conversations occurring in my head. I pretended the thoughts didn't exist. I had my successful moments. But many times I failed.

The next year, a series of recurring nightmares began. Always the dream would start with me walking out into a lake of water holding a baby in my arms. It was such a peaceful joyful moment. Then the dream would end tragically with the baby slipping through my arms. I saw the baby sinking down, down into the water.

I tried to reach it, but always its tiny fingers were just beyond my grasp. I looked down into the dark water to see the baby slowing sinking and then the baby's reflection in the water was forever gone. I would awake from the dream sobbing with tears. I had dropped my baby. I stood helplessly and watched as my baby sank to the bottom out of my grasp. The dream would haunt me for weeks afterwards.

Sometimes I would be exhausted and unable to sleep for fear the dream would come again. Always, I would go into a deep depression after the dream. In the next few years, the bouts with depression increased, along with this same recurring nightmare that many times caused me to dread going to sleep at night.

The dream continued quite frequently for another 7 years. Sometimes what I describe as a "heavy cloud" that I couldn't shake would hang over me. I felt like crying but the tears wouldn't come. I realize now, with all my therapy training that this was my way to process the pain of a loss that I had never allowed myself to grieve.

In retrospect, I believe if I had access to a book like *"C.P.R."*, if I would have had a venue to grieve and talk, these dreams would have stopped, I would have reached resolution at a much faster pace. Instead, I was isolated with no place to help me with the grief. I now realize so many other women were or are at this same place I was. What a shame!

You see, I didn't feel like I had the right to grieve my loss --there was no external evidence of a baby… and I didn't feel like I should be allowed permission to grieve over a loss that I had chosen.

My training now helps me understand that as human beings ALL losses must be grieved. Think of how, as a child, you began learning the grieving process. Oh, how painful it was to lose a friend or to lose that important ballgame. The loss of that first love…how painful is THAT! Even now as a parent, what a grief it was when my two boys walked out of the door to go to college! If you sit and think about life, look at how much loss is involved in the progression of life's daily living. Life is one long process of surviving and gaining victory in the midst of our losses.

Yet women who choose "vpt" are not allowed to cry about their loss, not even permitted by themselves, much less by other people. It is "expected" that we just "get on" with our lives. We are for the most part able to do that well.

At some point I went to a professional therapist in a town 180 miles away from me. I did want to ask him if the recurring dreams could be connected to the "vpt." I did not want anyone in my near vicinity to know about the choice I'd made so long ago, so I was forced to drive this distance to find someone who did not know me. Little did I realize that because of confidentiality protection laws, my information would not have been disclosed anyway! Again, so sad…we have "back door voluntary termination of pregnancy solutions" removed from our culture, but *resolution* for the grief surrounding the choice is still being accomplished "under cover." I drove 180 miles out of fear of disclosure in my local area concerning my deep, dark secret. This is a sad commentary on the disservice to women in our culture concerning choice decisions.

When I came clean to the therapist about the "vpt" and asked him about the dreams, he said, "You have made a valid choice. It is legal. You are making a big deal out of this. You need to just go home and get over it!" This was a total invalidation of my emotions by a professional. There is no way he understood that I was experiencing the effects of years of unresolved grief. I didn't need him to validate my choice; I needed him to validate my *grief!*

I went home and "limped along" for seven more long years. I struggled with the dreams, tried to push them away and went through the emotions of "doing life." Sometime later, in talking with a friend of mine who was a former pastor we somehow got on the topic of choice. His tone changed when he said, "I don't feel a bit sorry for those women. They kill their babies... they should feel bad!" This confirmed to me that I could never be too cautious about where my secret might slip out. I could never be safe in disclosing.

I continued to keep my secret well under wraps. Sometimes I would wake up crying in the night. However, I even learned to muffle the tears there. If my husband were home in bed with me he would get really angry. Even though I didn't "plan the tears" and really had no control over when I would just wake up crying, in frustration he would demand, "What are you crying about again?" I wouldn't realize until some years later, again while in training for grief counseling, that this "midnight crying" was my mind, heart and soul's way to process the grief I was feeling. Truly, the body remembers what the mind can't confess.

Eventually, I started going to a church where the pastor had an "I'm a Pro-Choice Pastor" as a bumper sticker on his car. I felt I would be "safe" here. Ironically, though, even this point of view did not validate me. The grief was there and the fact that he believed in choice almost made me feel crazier!

Why should I feel so bad if even my pastor was OK with my "vpt" decision? Sometimes even getting the choice confirmed can be invalidating as far as the sadness and grief that is still lingering deep inside.

"GO HOME AND GET OVER IT"

In my journey, I'd found three outlets for "help." One therapist and one pastor validated my choice, but not my *grief*. One pastor brought a message of condemnation and no hope. Truly, I had fallen through the cracks. I began to think I was the only person in the world with "this problem." I was alone with no one to throw me a life preserver. And the dreams continued. Finally, I met another person who had walked the valley of grief over "vpt." She gave me permission to cry. And cry I did. What a relief! What a difference that made in my life. I will be eternally grateful for this sister who walked me through the healing process.

So now I hope you see why it is so important that you know that you are NOT alone! There are others searching for answers. The crack is wide and the hole is deep. I hope this model of processing your choice will bring you the much needed resolution and validation you've been looking for!

What started as my own journey to peace has gone full circle. I've received my certificate of chaplaincy so I could learn how to counsel people in deep grief. I've gone through 12 long years of schooling to obtain my professional licensure in therapy. Now here I am …a professional person bringing the message of processing and resolution to the world. I am motivated to bring a new level of information to those suffering in silence with their secret.

I hope you'll be encouraged as we walk this road together.

The life raft is floating by your side. Hold on and know that you are being pulled to safety by someone who has been there holding onto the rope herself.

There is an ancient Chinese proverb, "When the student is ready, the teacher will come." It is no accident that you are reading this book. Your teacher is here so that means you are ready! Be encouraged and hopeful. You have permission to cry.

What I was feeling and what other women with a history of "vpt" are experiencing is something called *disenfranchised grief.* The word disenfranchised means to "deprive of a legal right, or of some privilege or immunity."

"My grief lies all within. And these external matters of lament are merely shadows to the unseen grief that swells with silence in the tortured soul."
W. Shakespeare, *The Tragedy of King Richard the Second*

"Oh the joy of comforting others in their time of need…to bring them bouquets of roses to refresh their languishing spirit!"
Trudy M. Johnson~my life mission!

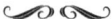

3

"Vpt" and Grief - It's Disenfranchised

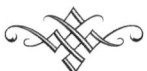

As we begin this chapter about grief, I would like to share this comment I found on the Internet by Rabbi Joshua L. Liebman: "Not only should we be unashamed of grief, confident that its expression will not permanently hurt us, but we should also possess the wisdom to talk about our loss and through that creative conversation with friends and companions begin to reconstruct the broken fragments of our lives… We should learn not to grow impatient with the slow healing process of time… We should anticipate these stages in our emotional convalescence: unbearable pain, poignant grief, empty days, resistance to consolation, disinterestedness in life, gradually giving way under the healing sunlight of love…"

For the person caught up in the wrangling of trying to resolve "vpt" there is only one small problem. We *are ashamed*. We feel shame when we think about sharing, talking about our choice. Since there is confusion about "vpt" being legal and therefore nothing to be grieved, our natural propensity is to feel ashamed to express sadness about a loss that we ourselves chose. It is a double whammy. Society says that everything about choice is fine but the challenge is, we feel alone and wonder if we are *not* "OK" because we are feeling a deep sense of sadness in our hearts. We feel sad. The world says we shouldn't feel sad. We should feel just fine. The confusing point therefore is the fact that our culture dismisses the natural occurrence of grief that is connected with a choice decision. It's *legal* therefore I am not allowed to feel sad. We are, unfortunately, comparing apples and oranges.

We are not only shamed because of the event…we should be getting on with our lives! We are ashamed of expressing grief about "vpt" to anyone for fear of condemnation or invalidation. Because there is no venue in which to talk about or acknowledge any loss attached to a voluntary pregnancy termination we are pretty much forced to stay silent.

Staying silent keeps us safe, but it doesn't stop the grief. I remember the times in my life when I spent dark moments wondering why I was sad, not knowing why I was sad, yet suspecting that this sadness was connected to my "vpt." Again, there was no one to talk to. When I did get the courage to do so, I got slammed down to the ground. I was invalidated by pro-choice people with an answer of "your choice was legal, you shouldn't feel bad. Go home and get over 'it.'"

I was invalidated by a the "other side." "You should feel bad, you killed your baby." I was stuck in the middle wondering who I could talk to. I honestly thought I was the *only one* on the face of the earth having these fuzzy feelings. I pushed them away, I pushed them down. I just didn't "go there." The only way to describe this place I was in was like living with a low-grade fever. Deep inside it felt like something was amiss, out-of-whack, not right. I wasn't sick, yet I wasn't 100% well. I was suspended in time. Not completely engaged in life, but still alive.

I didn't know I needed permission to grieve my loss. If I couldn't get permission from another human being, I needed permission to go through the grieving process from *myself*. This "vpt" journey I was on was my own solitary journey. Once you choose, it is no longer a political issue. It was no longer about being responsible or being irresponsible. This was about the sadness I needed to acknowledge because of my "vpt" choice.

Once I was given permission to grieve, a huge weight was lifted from my shoulders. It was hard walking the valley of grief, but the end result was peace.

Grief can be defined in many ways but in the case of "vpt" grief…the feelings are more like an unexplainable sadness or sorrow that hangs over us like a smoky cloud. There are no real definite descriptions. Every client and I…we all try to describe "the feeling." The descriptions are as varied as our own unique experiences. Yet the general idea of the feeling is complete common ground for us all.

There is just "something there" hanging out, lurking around, peeking around the corner in the shadows. This kind of grief is a pain that nags at the most inopportune times. It is a fruitless longing over something that you just can't quite put your finger on. It comes upon us, then goes away. Who knows what will "bring on" this mysterious feeling deep inside. Maybe it's the glimpse of a child. Maybe it's the change of seasons…the chill in the air…a summer's breeze…all depending upon the time in our past that the "vpt" occurred. For me, I always had a difficult time with mother's day. I never knew why. My children were awesome on this day for me. They showered me with wonderful love and affection. Yet on "this day" I found myself weepy and depressed. I would fight the feeling and try to appear happy. Deep inside, though, the blackness crept in.

I didn't realize until I began studying grief in my chaplaincy program that there are several types of grief. What I was feeling and what other women with a history of "vpt" are experiencing is something called *disenfranchised grief.* The word disenfranchised means to "deprive of a legal right, or of some privilege or immunity."[1] Isn't it interesting that we are given the right to legal termination of a pregnancy but we are not given the right to grieve the loss of the pregnancy when the time comes for us to do so.

As someone who made a choice in a difficult situation, I know the pain of "not being allowed to grieve" my loss. The grief is there but we do not give ourselves permission to "go there." Imagine that getting license to cry could actually be a *privilege!*

Again, the circumstances that might set the deep, dark feeling of grief in motion are varied. The actual word of the procedure… well, I avoided that like the plague. I always hated news stories that came on. I didn't want to hear "the word." I didn't want to think, hear or talk about IT.

However, hearing the word and seeing reminders of "the word" are pretty hard to avoid in the real world. In addition, seeing children, baby clothes, pregnant ladies, tiny wee ones being carried or in strollers…these things are what we see on a daily basis. Of course, even our own subsequent children are obvious realities before us.

And then there are all the revelations that are occurring rapidly through the miracles of science. Through ultrasound procedures, technology validates (as many of us have seen) evidence of our pregnancy loss.

Bottom line, what we all need to come face to face with as much as it jolts, hurts or makes us feel uncomfortable, is that in spite of our *reasons* for the choices we've made, it is an undeniable fact that we lost a pregnancy. In all likelihood every person reading this book right now (unless you are reading this to know about "vpt" to

---

1 Merriam-Webster Online Dictionary www.merriam-webster.com

understand a loved one), has experienced a pregnancy loss. There was a pregnancy there. Now it is gone. There is no proof or any confirmation of that pregnancy, but it all comes down to the fact that we went into a building one day somewhere in the world. When we came out, we were not pregnant.

A "vpt" experience does not erase the fact of pregnancy in our lives. The pregnancy will always be there…somewhere deep in our hearts…It is impossible to forget that we were "once pregnant" even if that pregnancy existed for just a short while.

Grief and guilt are natural reactions to pregnancy loss and ten times more for the "vpt" woman as opposed to a miscarriage event. At some point down the line after pregnancy loss there will rise up within a woman, pangs of guilt (possibly) and pains of grief absolutely!

Time out…let me qualify that the events of miscarriage and "vpt" are *totally* different. I would never want to compare these two situations nor even suggest they are similar. However, the internal hurt, pain and invalidation from the world can be very similar. For *both* miscarriage and "vpt" the grief and the guilt are there. The difference is that in cases of miscarriage *the guilt and grief are immediate* and are resolved in peace usually at least five years past the miscarriage event.

For "vpt" the immediate reaction typically is *relief. The guilt and grief do not creep out until many years later.* Ultimately, a place of resolution and peace may never be obtained unless that person finds a "teacher" to help them through.

Again, this grief usually does not surface until many years later. Typically, for the ladies I work with it is anywhere from 18-25 years *post "vpt."* As women go through their lives there comes a time when something called "a trigger" will put her in a place of grief concerning her "vpt."

C.P.R.

Those triggers can be other children about the same age, pregnant ladies, the actual word on news casts and verbal communications, or even seasonal changes that relate to the time of year the "vpt" occurred.

Besides ultrasound technology, research done in the area of stem cell science also points to why women do not forget their pregnancies. In an article printed by the American Academy of Pediatrics, Dr. Anne Stevens, MD, PhD and J. Lee Nelson, MD recount this amazing news: "It is now recognized that cells traffic between fetus and mother during pregnancy. Fetal cells have been found to persist for years, probably for a lifetime, in the circulation of normal women. Fetal cells pass into the maternal circulation during normal human pregnancy. Fetal microchimerism (the name of this process) during pregnancy is detected most readily in plasma and increases progressively over the course of gestation. Evidence of fetal cells in the mother's circulation has been described as early as 4 to 5 weeks of gestation."[2] This is a fancy way to say that "vpt" stops the pregnancy, but it doesn't stop the connection with that pregnancy. Literally, cells from the fetus come into our bodies and we carry them with us the rest of our days!

A connection this permanent deserves a grief process. We are not crazy! Deep inside we know we've experienced loss. It is ludicrous not to allow us to feel the pain of the loss at some point, when we are ready.

The evidence of loss is inside us. The evidence of loss is around us. Yet we sit in silence with "no right" to talk about or grieve that loss.

---

2 *"Maternal and Fetal Microchimerism: Implications for Human Diseases"* by Anne Stevens, MD, PhD and J. Lee Nelson, MD, NeoReviews, Vol3 No.1 2002, American Academy of Pediatrics.

For this reason, dear reader, rest assured you have a listening ear right now. I understand that your grief is real and that it must be acknowledged and validated. You have lost a pregnancy. You should be granted permission to grieve that loss. Once and for all let us separate Supreme Court legalities from the heart's normal and real cry to acknowledge pain and loss. Just know that there are so many others like you. We walk this path together and we cry the healing tears.

"Tears have a wisdom all their own. They come when a person has relaxed enough to let go and to work through his sorrow. They are a natural bleeding of an emotional wound, carrying the poison out of the system. Here lies the road to recovery." – F. Alexander Magoun

Important Suggestions Before We Begin:

As we walk this journey together, it is so important that you decide to be in charge of your own safety. I hope by now you have created that safe corner, nook, cranny, chair or any other place in your domain where you can sit and feel very safe. No matter how you have to decorate your space so that it *exudes* safety, please do so!

Again, include anything that will engage your five senses, whether it is a scented candle, music, pictures of loved ones, pictures of your favorite flowers, your favorite pet, soft "blankees"…anything and everything that will help you feel safe as we talk about the grief you might feel over your "vpt" decision.

Use this time of reflection to be "extra-nice" to yourself. Remember that you are *not alone* as you go into these unchartered waters. Somewhere across your town, across the state, across the country or even in the world, there is another woman, making her place of safety where she can begin her journey of processing and resolving her "vpt" loss. She, like you, is calling upon every ounce of internal courage she has.

Here are other tips for grieving loss:
1) Take care of yourself as you walk this journey. Processing the event might take a lot of emotional and even physical energy. Therefore, make sure you are treating yourself well during this time. Begin by trying to stay on track with your diet. Eating healthy food will keep you strong. Many of us medicate pain with our eating habits. Another helpful thing will be exercise. Exercise has proven to be one of the most helpful treatments for depression and stress. Exercising while you are dealing with difficult emotions will help you stay balanced and keep you from falling into depression.

2) Everyone grieves differently. Anne Morrow Lindbergh (who lost a child through his death because of a kidnapping) once said, "Grief can't be shared. Everyone carries it alone, his own burden, his own way." Responses to grief are as unique to individuals as fingerprints. Don't be hard on yourself if you take longer than anticipated. Don't be hard on yourself if you have a hard time crying or feeling any emotion. In other words, don't put this one in a box! Your unique grieving journey is yours. Just know that time is on your side and the more you get into the process and just "let it be" the brighter the sun will shine when you come through the other side of the tunnel. Sara Paddison, author of *Hidden Power of the Heart* says it best: "Some are able to release grief far more quickly than others. However long it takes, it is always the re-connection with the power of the heart that moves you past grief. When the heart is enlivened again, it feels like the

sun coming out after a week of rainy days. There is hope in the heart that chases the clouds away. Hope is a higher heart frequency and as you begin to reconnect with your heart, hope is waiting to show you new possibilities and the arrest of the downward spiral of grief and loneliness."[3]

3) Your body will never lie to you. You may experience difficulty sleeping during this time of "vpt" resolution. Don't eat or drink caffeine, drink alcohol, or exercise within 4-6 hours of bedtime. All of these things can make you feel better at first but will in the long run interrupt your sleep at night.

4) Any kind of herbal tea that is sleep-inducing can be your new best friend. A hot cup of chamomile tea right before bedtime can be very helpful.

5) A hot bath before bed is also a great way to help you relax before you crawl in. Usually you should do this at least an hour before bedtime. If you add Epsom salts to the water, it will have a wonderful calming effect - a cheap and safe way to relax stressed muscles, minds and hearts.

6) Support from others is important but not absolutely necessary. I get many questions like, "Should I tell my significant other I am going through 'C.P.R.'?" Of course, it depends. Is your relationship really secure? Is your S/O your best friend? As long as the person you tell is 100% supportive it won't hurt to have as many people encouraging you as possible. If you are like many, many clients of mine as well as myself, I was

---

3 *Hidden Power of the Heart*, Sara Paddison Out of Print but available from www.amazon.com

my sole cheerleader. It was a solitary journey for me. And that is why I hope this book will be an invaluable tool to help you along. I remind you again that you are not alone! Others are reading this same book today at the same time you are reading it. You can rest assured that you are not alone in this journey and that I am here walking beside you in your pain. We have different stories; we've handled the pain in different ways, but the emotional undercurrents we both feel are the same. You are not alone, so just make sure that anyone with whom you share that you are doing "this" will not have an invalidating answer or attitude. The goal is 100% safety…whatever that looks like for your individual situation!

I hope I am that safe person for you! I won't be telling you how to exactly walk out your "vpt" journey of grief. I just share my story and walk beside you to help you extract your story that's been tucked away for so long.

What's the Big Deal? What is there to Grieve?

We need to examine just what exactly our "vpt" losses were. Obviously, we weren't "ready" for a pregnancy at this stage in our life. So, we are not grieving decisions, but we do need to grieve the "other road" we didn't travel. Here are some possible losses attached to a "vpt."

1) Loss of the pregnancy. Births of subsequent children remind us that sometime in the past we had another pregnancy. So grieving the pregnancy is a very valid grief. Children and grandchildren are reminders of a pregnancy, long, long ago

in our lives. Again, as discussed earlier, "vpt" is a pregnancy loss. We need to accept the fact that we had a pregnancy that was not complete. Something natural was stopped. This loss creates a valid grief.

2) Loss of relationship. In general, most couples who are involved in a "vpt" will ultimately break up. Perhaps there is a person out there you thought would always be there for you. Now he is gone, too. Maybe he even left before the "vpt" or right afterwards. Maybe you chose "vpt" so you "wouldn't lose him." Yet even your "vpt" wasn't enough to make him stay. There is a list of loss of relationship surrounding "vpt" choices. Maybe you've lost other relationships when you shared your secret. Maybe you kept the secret in future relationships for fear of being discovered and dumped again. Especially you want to escape being judged or even condemned from yet another partner who might not understand your situation at the time of your choice.

For married partners, the grief of "vpt" affects the man and the woman differently. Your husband may completely minimize the pain you are feeling. Again there can be a lot of relationship conflicts because of "vpt" and the accompanying grief that can end up being unrecognized by a partner.

3) Loss of dreams. Maybe the "vpt" was something you weren't really in control of. Maybe you were pressured by your partner, by your parents or in the case of medical "vpt," by a doctor. Maybe you really felt like there was no other way "out" of your crisis. Maybe you didn't get another chance at

pregnancy so you are really feeling guilty about your "vpt" choice. I've worked with many ladies who were eventually not able to get pregnant when the time became right. This can be very painful for women in this place of grief. They are grieving not only the "vpt" but they are also grieving the loss of ever being pregnant again. Another double whammy!

4) Loss of control. In a world where we want to be in command and in charge of perfection, we can think back on the "vpt" and cringe. It's a constant reminder that we weren't always in control. We thought the choice would bring even more control. The "vpt" is the secret we have to keep so that we can keep the façade going that we are perfect. Keeping the illusion of perfection going can be very exhausting. As we process our "vpt" decision we all need to stop beating ourselves up about perfection. Perfection is really a mindset that we need to ditch if we are ever to find peace.

As you can see, the pregnancy isn't the only thing that needs to be grieved. There are other elements connected to the "vpt" choice that weave through our minds and hearts. Keeping the secret uses up a lot of emotional energy. We start thinking differently about ourselves, others and the world. For "vpt" there is nowhere to go to process the experience. If only there were some sort of safe place to share!

The turmoil keeps going inside, the emotions float around unidentified. The losses beg to be acknowledged and cried over. No measure of logic ("why don't I just get over this?") will bring peace like recognizing the losses in a truthful way and giving ourselves the incredibly healing permission to grieve a "vpt."

"VPT" AND GRIEF - IT'S DISENFRANCHISED

Loss not grieved turns to sorrow in our heart. That sorrow manifests itself as depression or anger. Acceptance precedes change. Accepting that your "vpt" was a pregnancy loss will give you the permission you need to let yourself "go there" in your grief.

Truth can be very freeing. Acknowledging the pain of loss surrounding your "vpt" choice will bring a relief to your heart that you may not at this time actually understand. As painful as this process is, rest assured you are not alone in your pain and the sun is shining at the end of your path!

Identifying the Core Grief Issues

According to Elizabeth Kubler-Ross, there are five stages of grief. Denial is the first stage of grief, followed by bargaining, anger, depression and finally acceptance. For those of us who haven't been allowed to grieve a "vpt" we can stay stuck in anger and not even realize why we are so angry. The anger might manifest itself as depression. This usually is a low level of depression. Not connecting that depression to unprocessed grief concerning a "vpt" decision is typical. You see, because there is such a taboo, disconnect or ignorance (whichever label you want to put on it) concerning permission to grieve a "vpt" we try to go straight to "acceptance", thus bypassing a few of the steps in the grieving process." The acceptance stage works for awhile. We stay in acceptance by using the coping skill of denial. We spend years denying that nagging heart's voice to cry about voluntary pregnancy termination. Denial is our friend. It works very well as we try to move to acceptance. In between, though, anger and depression may lurk in the background. This is typically described as an unidentifiable feeling that can't really be explained. The "vpt" woman "just knows" *something* uncomfortable is living inside them. Denial protects from the pain.

C.P.R.

The "key" to *really* going to true acceptance is working through the grief process. For women of choice, this is a bit hard. Society says there is *nothing to grieve*. We tell ourselves we are glad we had the right to choice. Once again, there is a disconnect between *the right to choose* and *the right to grieve*. Right to choose does not wipe out our loss. Confusing the legalities with permission to engage our hearts in a normal human process, grieving, is what causes so much guilt and shame, anger and depression for the woman of choice. It is this point we will begin the first stage of moving from denial *through the pain of the grief process* onto the acceptance stage of the grieving process. It is simply *not normal* to try to reach acceptance straight away.

I want to make sure you understand, my "vpt sister," that moving from denial into the grief stage can be a very painful step. This will take a lot of courage for you. Please understand that others are holding their breath like you right now. Please go to your "safe place," comfort yourself, wrap up in your blankee as we take this first step of grieving by digging deeper into your heart to access the emotions of grief that lay there in the darkness. Rest assured it is this process of going towards the darkness that will bring you out into the light of closure.

You are not alone! You, me, the sisterhood is here! We understand your fear. We celebrate your courage as you identify what exactly it is that you need to grieve. You will use this Grief Worksheet to identify all the losses that surround your voluntary pregnancy choice.

I have included three worksheets in this section. The multiple worksheets are for those dear ones who have more than one "vpt" to process. If you need more than three worksheets, feel free to make copies of these for further use.

Again, stay safe as you tackle this first step of moving from denial to processing.

"VPT" AND GRIEF - IT'S DISENFRANCHISED

The challenge for "vpt" is that it "feels like" denial helps us go down the straight path to acceptance. In reality, we are by-passing part of the grieving process steps with resulting "low grade" fevers of anger and depression. Staying in denial about your loss will never bring you out to the other side of resolution. If you by-pass connecting in your emotions with your loss, you will stay stuck in anger or suppressed anger (depression) the rest of your days. If you deny *what* you lost, you will never *accept* that loss deep within your heart.

∽∾

To avoid writing in this book, copying any worksheet exercises in "C.P.R." is permitted by the author.

C.P.R.

My Grief Worksheet

Possible losses you might recognize:

Pregnancy, relationship (parents, boyfriend, etc), loss of control,

loss of dreams

Identify your loss	I need to forgive myself?	I need to forgive someone? Who?	I've felt the pain of this loss?

My Grief Worksheet

Possible losses you might recognize:

Pregnancy, relationship (parents, boyfriend, etc), loss of control, loss of dreams

Identify your loss	I need to forgive myself?	I need to forgive someone? Who?	I've felt the pain of this loss?

C.P.R.

My Grief Worksheet

Possible losses you might recognize:

Pregnancy, relationship (parents, boyfriend, etc), loss of control,

loss of dreams

Identify your loss	I need to forgive myself?	I need to forgive someone? Who?	I've felt the pain of this loss?

NOTES:

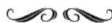

Emotions are like children. They want attention.
They don't want to be ignored.

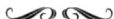

Grieving the losses and labeling the emotions you feel about a
"vpt" are ways to free you up in other areas of your life.

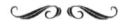

As you start this process, if you find yourself getting
overwhelmed you are permitted to stop and just sit and relax and
listen to your music and be still. If you find yourself getting too
emotional to concentrate you are permitted to stop the process
anytime you want. You do have control over whether or not you
proceed with processing.

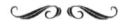

4

I Second that Emotion

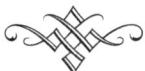

As you read this chapter you will experience many different emotions. It is important that you stay safe while you let yourself go to those emotions. Since your "vpt" is probably an event that you've stored away in your mind it is possible that you really haven't attached any emotions to the situation you were in at the time you made the decision. For the most part, we've all been in a place of just ignoring or numbing any emotion attached to making a decision for choice.

Unresolved grief can actually cause emotions deep within that we do not consciously relate to an actual event. Because there is no venue in which to talk about or acknowledge any loss attached to a voluntary pregnancy termination we are pretty much forced to store those emotions deep inside.

Try to think about sitting in a room talking with a friend. Say flames start bursting through the heating duct in the ceiling above your head. Imagine your voice continues on. You are calm as you describe the beautiful ocean side where you recently went on vacation. Your friend listens and laughs as you talk joyfully about the wonderful time you had on the beach. Smoke fills the room, yet you continue to serenely ignore your surroundings. On the inside you are starting to be fearful. You think maybe you should run or scream. Yet, you keep your composure. Your friend listens while you continue to visit nonchalantly. Internally you know that "things aren't right" but externally you display a great measure of calm. You hold it all together while the whole building becomes engulfed in flames. You are good at seeming "fine" so instead of now throwing a chair at the window and escaping through the broken glass, you finish your dialogue with sublime composure. This is what happens when we have unprocessed emotions screaming to be heard. We can appear together, but internally we know that we are dangerously close to combusting into flames or suffocating in the black smoke.

It's been said that emotions are a bit like little children tugging at your skirt. They want you to notice them. They want your attention. You have some emotions that have been pushed down for perhaps years now. You are permitted in this safe venue to reach down and attach a name to each emotion that wants recognition. You know how a child will "shut up" when you stop everything and pay attention to "just them." So it is with your emotions. Once you recognize them, put labels to them, they won't carry the passion…they won't keep knocking on your door to be recognized. Like a child being rocked to sleep, these emotions will rest and cause no more noise deep within your soul. Now is your time to acknowledge what you are feeling concerning the day you chose to voluntarily terminate your pregnancy and the days, months and years afterwards.

You probably haven't ever had anyone ask *how you felt on that day*. The emotions are there. They just need permission to come out. What you need to know is that processing this part of the grief you feel is probably the hardest step. Letting yourself feel the emotion can be very uncomfortable. You've spent a lifetime or at least several years avoiding what you felt. Now to turn and go in the direction of acknowledging how you felt…that can be scary and make you feel uneasy. When you try on a new pair of shoes they don't often feel right at first. Sometimes they "take some getting used to." So it is when you actually attach emotion to your voluntary pregnancy termination experience. *Feeling,* after all, was not permitted until now. It is often hard to "go there" when it's such a foreign concept. Additionally, please know that the common emotion that is going to surface is anger. Anger at yourself, anger at others…anger, anger, anger!

If anger is the first emotion that comes out as we do this exercise, then you are not going deep enough into the grief. You see, anger is a *secondary* emotion. Anger is the emotion we are allowed to express, both in our present culture and in our general humanness. But anger is not the *primary* emotion you are feeling. What comes out as anger is really about hurt, unmet expectations or unmet needs. When it comes to "vpt" these emotions can be directed at ourselves or others or both. So, if you answer anger, you are not digging deep enough into your emotions. We have to go deeper to get to the bottom of the grief.

As we start looking at some of these emotions then, it could be that you will start to feel angry. Again, the anger isn't *really* what you are feeling. It is for this reason you need to understand that this chapter which is aimed at identifying the emotions you feel as a result of your "vpt" is probably the hardest part of your journey. This is why it is so important for you to have peace and comfort while you are in this part of processing a "vpt."

Again, it is advised that you be in a safe environment, your "safe place" to read this book. I hope you have a quiet place that brings stillness to your soul. Perhaps you have a candle lit, some soft music playing and you even might have your "blankee" covering your lap. Going into those emotions from a place of comfort is very important. As you read it is also important for you to know that you are not alone. Even if for all appearances, you are the only one dealing with your "vpt," know that first of all there are other ladies reading this book exactly like you are. Also know the author had to tackle the scary thing of attaching emotion to her "vpt" event. Believe me, it was really hard for me when I first started working through this. I didn't realize how compacted the emotion was that I was feeling. I had buried the emotions very deep. I was unaware of the fact that buried emotions *don't die*. They just lie there rotting, stinking, causing more harm.

There are actually physiological changes that happen to the brain when we have emotions in us that we haven't dealt with. These emotions are stored in the right side of the brain. Being in a physical place that exudes warmth, comfort and serenity will engage the right side of your brain. Appealing to the right side of your brain will help those stuck emotions to get pried loose so that you can pick them up, handle them and eventually give them a place of peaceful rest. Anything that involves the five senses will help unlock that right-brain place. Scented candles (smell and soft light), soft blankets (touch) and soft music (hearing) all contribute to thawing the emotions you've locked away in the right side of your cranial cavity---your brain.

If you've not accessed the emotions related to your "vpt" then at first you may just say, "I feel nothing about it or I am just numb." Did you know that "numb" is actually an emotion? So even if the only thing you can pull out is "numb" or "angry" you are still accessing some sort of emotional response to a past "vpt." This is our starting place. Look at the process as a horizontal line. On one end you have "numb" or no emotion. On the other end of the line we will put "anger." It is at the points in between where the pain of grief lies.

What's so necessary about identifying the emotion connected to a "vpt" you say? The importance of recognizing those emotions is that our emotions do not occur in a vacuum. If you are "numbing out" emotions related to a pregnancy termination you will also "numb out" emotions in relationships that require a deep level of connection.

Flat-lining one event will cause other important events in your life to also be flat-lined or dead. For example, if anger over a "vpt" is present then you might also express anger towards yourself and/ or others in other important areas of your life. That anger can either be displayed as outside anger (rage…being angry at a level that doesn't match the event) or it can go inside and manifest itself as depression.

So I hope you see that stuffed down emotions about a "vpt" will eventually start affecting other relationships and behavioral reactions in your life. Unbeknownst to you, the road rage you feel when driving the freeway might actually be a way for you to release the anger you feel towards yourself or others in regard to the "vpt" in your past.

As mentioned earlier, grief connected to a "vpt" is what we call *disenfranchised* grief. Disenfranchised grief is grief we don't permit ourselves to experience. Disenfranchised grief eventually leads to *displaced* anger. We can display anger over a seemingly innocent action or event. Basically, we can use anger to punish to a much higher level than the crime deserves.

Grieving the losses and labeling the emotions you feel about a "vpt" are ways to free you up in other areas of your life. For so many ladies I've worked with (and also for myself) there existed a much lower level of anger (volatile and depression) after processing a past "vpt."

Here are some ways in which not connecting with the emotion

around a "vpt" might be affecting you. I myself experienced *all* of these symptoms. You may not be in the same place I was, but it is pretty certain that you are dealing with at least one or two of the following listings because of your unresolved "vpt" choice.

- Intense feelings of guilt
- Thoughts of suicide or preoccupation with death
- Feelings of worthlessness
- Life detached behavior – appearing disconnected from the present
- Inability to function with daily tasks (home, school, work)
- Complete loss of pleasure in previously enjoyed events

Do you find yourself dealing with intense guilt about your "vpt?" Perhaps you do not realize that unprocessed grief can cause a person to feel guilty. Jerry Sittser once said in *A Grace Disguised*, "Regret keeps wounds of loss from healing, putting us in a perpetual state of guilt."

You see, what happens to many of us is that when we were in that tough place of having to "choose," our lives were probably in complete chaos. Our choices were made in a state of crisis. I know I just wanted the crisis to be "over." I found the quickest and easiest solution.

Years down the road I was able to step back and look at my "vpt" choice. Now that I was in a different place … not only physically, but also emotionally, financially and mentally…I began to question and bounce back and forth. Again, there was no one to talk to about it---except myself!

If you bounce back and forth enough between the "what-if's" and "if-only's" you reach a place of exhaustive guilt. We analyze until we paralyze. We push away the emotion of it all and for small increments of time we seem to arrive at some measure of rest.

I SECOND THAT EMOTION

As hard as it is to go back to the little box in the right side of your brain that holds the recording of emotions you feel about a "vpt," it is necessary you do so. Prying the lid off that box will give you a new sense of freedom and peace that will affect other areas of your life including important connected relationships. It is "worth it" to go through the pain of facing the emotions head-on. What you can't talk about keeps you in bondage and comes out in other ways to bring you down.

Henry David Thoreau once said, "Each man interprets another's experience only by his own." This is why it is important that you have someone who has "been there" where you are right now to talk with you about the hidden, stuffed emotions from a past "vpt." You can take my experience with "vpt" and run yours through my grid. I think you will find that we've both walked the same road. This makes us kindred souls. I know the pain of keeping my secret for decades. I know the fear of sitting in the room that's engulfed in flames and wondering if the listener can see the panic on my face as I try to stay collected and calm. I know the frustration of not being able to talk and the angst of wondering if I was the only one feeling sadness. The daily dialogue of non-congruent thoughts became a prison I couldn't walk out of. Yet those around me marveled at my ability to be cool and collected. Keeping those emotions locked away with no one to discuss them with required more and more energy. Finding a safe place to open the box and let the emotions fly out…what a wonderful new world that was. So for you I encourage you to go through the pain and fear of opening up the lid to your stuffed away emotions. Going through that pain in this safe place is worth it for the freedom you will feel on the other side.

You must be willing to visit the place of personal grief to come out on the other side. Why does this sadness come upon us when we were so sure about our choice? It is important to look at life as a continually rolling documentary. A place we were in at the time of choice is not the place we are probably now living in.

As hard as it seems, dear one, you simply must go through this journey of facing the emotions you feel about your past "vpt" to process them and to reach a place of resolution and peace for the future. Thankfully, you do not have to go through the process alone. This book is here to assist you. Others are reading it just like you so rest assured you are not alone!

I am going to use a very effective tool to help you pull out the emotions you might be feeling concerning your "vpt." Remember identifying the emotion and then letting yourself feel that emotion is the way to put the emotions to rest.

Identifying "vpt" Emotions:

1) Talk about all the details you can remember.
2) Identify people involved in the event.
3) Identify the emotions attached to the event.
4) Identify the emotions attached to the people involved.
5) Using the feeling chart identify your emotions before, during and after the event.
6) Journal about the event, expressing all the emotion you've identified about the event and people, including yourself.

Pull the chain…get off the train!

As you start this process, if you find yourself getting overwhelmed you are permitted to stop and just sit and relax and listen to your music and be still. If you find yourself getting too angry to concentrate you are also permitted to stop the process anytime you want. You do have control over whether or not you proceed with processing.

I SECOND THAT EMOTION

Special Cases of Voluntary Pregnancy Termination "VPT" and Medical Decisions

If you terminated your pregnancy because of a medical diagnosis of adverse pregnancy, your situation is a little different than a person faced with an unplanned pregnancy. Just know that even though your circumstances were entirely different, the grief you feel is still disenfranchised grief that has no venue to grieve publically.

Adverse pregnancy diagnoses are very common. I once worked on a crisis line and many times the callers were those trying to decide what to do when they received a recommendation by their physician to terminate.

I do believe this special reason for a "vpt" choice can render even more grief and pain and mixed emotions. Usually, this pregnancy is a planned one or at the very least is in the confines of marriage. The circumstances are very different than say a fourteen year old girl who is pregnant. For this reason, there are many more components of questioning a "vpt" decision. The guilt and grief can be even stronger and more devastating.

These are tough, tough circumstances. I believe the invalidation for women put into these positions can be even more intense. The doctor who is a professional usually gives tremendous assurance of this being "the right thing to do." Therefore, there can be an implication that "you've done the right thing so why should you feel bad?" Again, a terribly intense form of disenfranchised grief!

Perhaps you are faced with even more "what-if's." "What-if" I had allowed the pregnancy in spite of the diagnosis?" "What if things would have turned out OK for my pregnancy? "What if the doctor was wrong?" You can beat yourself up with the "what-if's" for the rest of your life.

What will bring you closure, however, will be giving yourself permission to grieve your loss. Again, it is because you were in a position to make the choice that society does not expect you to grieve your loss. Still this is a loss and what you are feeling is disenfranchised grief.

You should go ahead and do all the exercises including the journaling. Again, understand that going back and forth with the "what-if's" is a futile exercise. It will not bring you peace, only more guilt and pain.

Use these exercises to work through the pain of your loss and just know that you are not alone. Others are out there who have also terminated pregnancies because of adverse diagnosis from doctors. The grief is the same because you have all lost a pregnancy.

"VPT" Decisions and Sexual Assault or Sexual Abuse

If you have chosen to voluntarily terminate a pregnancy either because of sexual assault or sexual abuse, you have even more pain to process. I highly recommend that you seek additional counseling for these issues. You might have high levels of anger, fear and shame that are influencing the way you feel. This author works with many of these types of special cases in her private practice and has found brief intensive therapy to be very helpful in these difficult situations. Read more at www.missingpieces. org. You can take a self-test here concerning your past sexual assault or abuse or trauma bond that occurred as a result of this life-altering event.

Just know that you also have permission to grieve the loss of your pregnancy. Even though you may feel an intense amount of guilt and shame regarding the circumstances of your "vpt" you still need to gain closure by grieving the loss you feel in your heart concerning your decision to terminate, regardless of the circumstance surrounding that choice.

Again, you can proceed through *"C.P.R."* just as any other woman who is processing her "vpt" choice. Focus on the grief and anger you feel as you work through the emotions and the journaling. You do have permission to grieve this loss. Even though you may feel like a victim, this is still a loss that needs to be grieved. You have permission. You are not alone! By the time a woman reaches the age of 18, one in three will have been sexually abused. You are not alone in your pain!

Grieving a "vpt" loss resulting from rape or sexual abuse is a way to move from the position of victim to a place of survivor and victory.

Multiple "vpt" Choices

Some statistics show that 55% of women who make a "vpt" decision will go on to make the same choice again, and 20% of those ladies will choose a third time. More and more among my clients, I am seeing multiple terminations. This is a common practice, so please do not think you are the only one. Actually, last year multiple "vpt's" was more the norm than the exception. The majority of the women I work with experience anywhere from three to six terminations. Again, do not think you are the only one when it comes to multiple "vpt" decisions.

While it may be a bit harder for you, I highly recommend that you work through the "vpt" choice that sticks out in your mind with the most clarity. Work through this one first before processing the others. It may seem overwhelming at first to think about processing all the choices. This is why you start with the one that had the most impact on your life or at least the one that you are most mindful of.

C.P.R.

When you feel you've received closure for that one, you may choose to do the others separately or together. The important thing is that you start the closure process. DO NOT let the fact that you have more than one to work through stop you! It will get easier as you go along. I remind you again that multiple "vpt" choices are very normal in our society. Each termination is deserving of closure.

Work through each "vpt" with patience and internal fortitude. Take a rest when you feel like you need it, but do continue on in the journey.

Sit quietly in your safe place, listen to your music, and quiet yourself. Realize this is a process and at first it might be hard to access all those emotions that have been pushed down for so long.

Up and out is how "it" works!

Letting the emotion come up and out is what is going to help you reach a point of resolution. As hard as it is, try to let those emotions out. If you need to cry, let yourself cry. At first it might be scary to let yourself cry. Sometimes it seems like if you start, you might not stop because the tears have been inside so long. However, just know that there will come an end to the tears. With the tears comes peace.

Unfortunately, it is necessary to go through the pain to the tears and then you will have peace. Don't get discouraged with the process. Everyone is on a different timetable for processing and resolving. Let yourself start and stop as many times as you need. As you go along, it will get easier and easier to identify and feel the emotions. Be patient with yourself. You are not on any schedule or timeline. You can go at the speed you need to go. Just let yourself feel again. Feel and cry until you have expressed all the emotion that's in there about your "vpt" choice.

Before you begin the exercise on the next page make sure you are feeling safe, comforted and protected. This is your time to cry.

I SECOND THAT EMOTION

You have permission to feel. You have permission to cry. Identify those emotions and get them up and out!

Basic Instructions

Before you begin filling out the *"VPT" Emotional Distresses Worksheet©* you might consider making copies of it. This will give you more flexibility to think about each emotion and also to write or doodle as you see fit. If you are reading this book in a library this leaves the book in proper order for the next person to use it.

C.P.R.

"VPT" Emotional Distresses Worksheet
LEVEL ONE

This worksheet has the 3 main negative emotions that humans experience.

<u>Try to identify just one main category of emotions for each event - before, during, after the "vpt."</u> At first you may find it confusing to pick out the *main emotion*. If you try really hard, though, you will see that one main emotion stands out more than the other two.

You will identify the *main* emotion for each question

BEFORE THE "VPT"	SAD	MAD	SCARED
Making the decision - my part made me feel…			
Parents' input made me feel…			
The thought of allowing my parents' input made me feel…			
Boyfriend's/husband's input made me feel…			
Friends made me feel…			
Others' input (if any) made me feel…			
DURING THE "VPT"			
I felt…			

I SECOND THAT EMOTION

	SAD	MAD	SCARED
IMMEDIATELY AFTER THE "VPT"			
I felt…			
Partner/husband made me feel…			
Friends made me feel…			
Others made me feel…			
RIGHT NOW			
I feel…			
Partner/husband makes me feel…			
Friends make me feel…			
Others make me feel…			

Notes:

C.P.R.

"VPT" Emotional Distresses Worksheet
LEVEL TWO

On the previous page you identified the main emotion attached to the event/person. Now, using the additional words on the second level, identify even deeper emotions. You will remain in the same column you chose in Level One, proceeding down to Level Two. You can select individual emotions or if you felt ALL of the 2nd level emotions, you can write "ALL" in the space provided.

	SAD	MAD	SCARED
Second Level Emotions	**Guilty, ashamed, depressed, lonely**	**Hurt, hostile, angry, rage, hateful, critical**	**Rejected, confused, helpless, submissive, insecure, anxious**
BEFORE THE "VPT"			
Making the decision - my part made me feel…			
Parents' input made me feel…			
The thought of allowing my parents' input made me feel…			
Boyfriend's/husband's input made me feel…			
Friends made me feel…			
Others' input (if any) made me feel…			
DURING THE "VPT"			

I SECOND THAT EMOTION

I felt…			
IMMEDIATELY AFTER THE "VPT"			
I felt…			
Partner/husband made me feel…			
Friends made me feel…			
Others made me feel…			
RIGHT NOW			
I feel…			
Partner/husband makes me feel…			
Friends make me feel…			
Others make me feel…			

C.P.R.

"VPT" Emotional Distresses Worksheet
LEVEL THREE

On the previous page you identified the 2nd level emotions attached to the event/person. Now, using the additional words on the third level, identify even deeper emotions. You will remain in the same column you chose in Level One, proceeding down to Level Three. You can select individual emotions or if you felt ALL of the 3rd level emotions, you can write "ALL" in the space provided.

	SAD	MAD	SCARED
Second Level Emotions	Guilty, ashamed, depressed, lonely	Hurt, hostile, angry, rage, hateful, critical	Rejected, confused, helpless, submissive, insecure, anxious
Third Level Emotions	**Apathetic, Inferior, Inadequate, Miserable, Stupid,**	**Jealous, Selfish, Frustrated, Furious, Irritated, Skeptical**	**Bewildered, Discouraged, Insignificant, Weak, Foolish, Embarrassed**
BEFORE THE "VPT"			
Making the decision - my part made me feel…			
Parents' input made me feel…			
The thought of allowing my parents' input made me feel…			
Boyfriend's/husband's input made me feel…			

I SECOND THAT EMOTION

Friends made me feel…			
Others' input (if any) made me feel…			
DURING THE "VPT"			
I felt…			
IMMEDIATELY AFTER THE "VPT"			
I felt…			
Partner/husband made me feel…			
Friends made me feel…			
Others made me feel…			
RIGHT NOW			
I feel…			
Partner/husband makes me feel…			
Friends make me feel…			
Others make me feel…			

"VPT" Distresses Worksheet Copyright 2010 Trudy M. Johnson
www.missingpieces.org

C.P.R.

Congratulations! Identifying these emotions has not been easy. Please take some time to look at your Emotional Distress Sheet. Did the majority of your emotions that you felt concerning your "vpt" fall into one category of emotion? Typically, this is the case. And if this is the case for you, look at all the emotions that pertain to your main emotion category. Are these the emotions you struggle with in your relationships? I hope you can see that these core feelings might be stemming from the fact that you have not processed grief relating to the "vpt" experience! NOW aren't you glad you've gone through the pain of these exercises? Doing so will help you have more victory in your life when feeling these emotional triggers.

If your emotions fell into more than one category, it is likely that you are having even more challenges with emotion regulation. Typically, you are either over-regulating your emotions by not allowing yourself to feel or you are under-regulating your emotions. This type of emotional pattern will result in over-reacting to things that require emotional fortitude. For example, you may appear to be a highly emotional person. The emotions you respond with in situations might be more volatile than a normal expression of emotions. You may explode in anger, or you may feel very weak and go into your shell when faced with an emotional trial. Again, I hope you can see that some of the reactions you've had in life might be connected to unprocessed grief surrounding your "vpt" experience!

The secret to gaining emotional freedom is to place labels on the emotions you are feeling. If you can do that you can begin to understand why you react the way you do and understand *why* you feel inadequate, weak, or hostile. Just the mere fact that you've now assigned labels to the emotions you are feeling over your "vpt" experience will bring you to a whole new level of peace. Part of the process of grieving means having a safe venue to tell your story and then identifying the emotions you feel because of the experience.

I SECOND THAT EMOTION

PERMISSION TO FEEL…GRANTED.

Here is an exercise you can work through to take those emotions out of your emotion box.

EMOTION BOX

Use this area to list the emotions you identified in the previous exercises.

Here are the main emotions I felt about my "vpt":

Go through each emotion. Practice recognizing that emotion. Practice feeling the pain of that emotion. Repeat this validation for each emotion you wrote.

"I have permission to feel the pain of _____."

(name of emotion)

I give this emotion permission to come out of the box. I have permission to feel this emotion. I have permission to cry when I feel the pain of this emotion. It is OK to cry."

Go through your "permission to feel" emotions several times as you allow yourself to feel them and allowing yourself to cry.

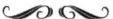

Staying in denial about grief delays the process
and prolongs the pain.

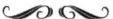

Acknowledging that grief exists brings freedom from
the bondage that grief creates.

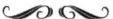

Be safe and know that you are not alone as you write!

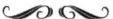

5

Beginning to Tell My Story

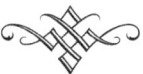

In this next section on grief you will begin sticking your toe into the dreaded lake of sorrow. Please know that you are going through this journey at your own speed. You are not under any pressure to accomplish this task in any timeframe.

Processing grief is accomplished at your own pace. This is your unique journey, your own special time and place. This process of reaching into your heart and opening a door that's been closed for so long will bring you a new sense of joy. Look upon this experience of permission to grieve your "vpt" loss as an opportunity! This exercise of "vpt" processing and resolution will move you out of the past and into the present.

Only you know the pace you need to keep. Maybe you want to swing the door to your heart right open and jump in. For others, you may want to turn the knob slowly, letting the latch unclick and then push the door open slightly. Whatever speed you need to go is your own unique journey.

For me, there was almost a decade of processing before I was able to make progress. That was partly because I didn't have a resource like this in front of me. I took one step forward and then some years, two steps back. It is my hope that *"C.P.R."* will spare you extra pain and accelerate this resolution process for you.

In the next chapter you will journal your own story. The process of recalling one's own story is very cathartic. Telling your story will bring power and closure to your life. Journaling your story will start at the beginning and progress all the way to the closing of the grief process. Somewhere in between you will find a new level of peace.

Although pain and grief are the things we avoid in our life, pain and grief are what make us who we are. We cannot reach completeness if we don't go through the pain. The hidden pain of "vpt" is the common bond of everyone working through this book right now. Again, may I say, "you are not alone!" Other women are on this same page right now. Some are dreading this part and are tempted to put the book down or even to skip over this part of the process. I would encourage you to try to persevere through the pain. Going through the pain is our "door of hope" for resolution and closure.

This process will help you see others and yourself in a different light. Pain shared is a common bond that brings us to a place in our souls that nothing else can. Walking this journey of pain will bring you through to the other side into a new place of peace and freedom. Ridding yourself of the grief you've been carrying in secret will renew your vigor. With this new level of freedom you will have enough energy left over to see other's pain in a more caring way.

Am I actually saying pain is a good thing? YES! The act of processing pain can be seen as a gift! Going through the pain to resolution will make you a different person. Pain resolved is a pain that is never wasted. Going through the journaling process will help you identify areas of lost emotions and thoughts that have been hidden away concerning your voluntary pregnancy termination.

BEGINNING TO TELL MY STORY

It is important that you stay safe while you express your thoughts about your voluntary pregnancy termination on paper. If you have a hard time journaling about your experience, you can try this. Go to the safe place you have created. Again, make sure you've processed some of those emotions in the previous chapter. Now it is time to take one more step towards closure. In the following pages you have permission to put the puzzle pieces of your own story together. It is my hope that you are treating yourself with care by lighting a candle, playing soft music, drinking a specialty tea. Now get a small alarm clock and set the clock for 20 minutes. You only have to write for 20 minutes. If you haven't thought of anything for 20 minutes, or maybe you just have a few sentences, stop the exercise and come back to it at a later time when you are ready. At any rate, you only have to write for 20 minutes. Setting this parameter will take the pressure off if you are afraid to start writing.

You can pick up your journal and put it down as often as you like. Just know that you have permission to write about your "vpt" and know that others are struggling to write their thoughts also. *You are not alone!* You have permission to write only a limited amount. As time passes you will allow yourself to write more and more until eventually you will feel comfortable letting the words fly out of your pen and onto the page.

Maybe you will be one of the fortunate few who won't need to set the alarm for 20 minutes! You might be able to write freely. Whatever works for you, this is the important thing.

Rather than write in this book, a suggestion would be for you to buy a nice journal that you can keep in an out of the way place. Journaling in a nice book with colored paper and a nice cover seems to make the process more appealing. Of course you may use this book if it belongs to you and I've made room on the pages for you to scribe your story if this is the place you choose. Writing in a nice journal type book though would be my suggestion.

Journaling Guidelines:

1) Patience is important! You are not being "graded" on what you write. This exercise is for you and you alone! Do not be pressured about how many words you are writing or if you are unable to express yourself very well. Hiding your "vpt" has been a lifelong experience for you. It might take a bit of patience to actually put words on the paper. This can not only feel uncomfortable, it can actually invoke downright fear. It will be "so freeing" once you get everything "up and out."

I help many of my clients understand this part of the process as the "vomit stage." Personally, I hate to throw up! I've been known to lie on the bed for hours trying to make the feeling go away. All this does is keep me sick. Once I get up and go "get it out" I feel *much* better.

You have been carrying "this" around for years. Getting it up and out will be essential for your resolution process!

2) Safety first! I know I keep reminding you to be in a safe place when you work through your *"C.P.R."* book. Again, I take the liberty of suggesting that you go to your safe spot to begin your writing. Also, choose a time when you won't be interrupted. For myself and many others I've worked with, it's been necessary to choose a very early morning time. This seems to be the time of day with fewest interruptions. If you are a "night owl" this would obviously be the best time

of day for you to start this journey. Whichever timeframe best fits into your personality type…use this time of day to write your "vpt" story.

Additionally, knowing what part of the day is the best time for you to settle down into quietness is part of knowing yourself. We are all so uniquely crafted and we all have a time of day that finds us the most quiet, most reflective and most creative. This is the time of day you need to choose to do your journaling. I would not recommend writing "just when you can fit it in." This journaling part of the process is too serious and too painful and too introspective for you to treat it as just another homework assignment for a class. You won't accomplish the closure necessary if you don't engage your heart in the process. Don't rush through. Put as much thought and emotion as possible into your writing. It needs to "flow" and be as honest and natural as possible. This is the type of writing that comes from the deep quietness of your heart, not the logical places of your brain.

3) Before you begin writing, try to think about the words coming from deep inside. You can even try picturing your heart. If you could find an object that represents what your heart looks like, what shape would it be? Would it be hard, prickly, sharp or soft? Picturing your words flowing out of your heart will help you write your true feelings. Again, if you start expressing what is in your head, this exercise will not be as helpful or as honest as it needs to be.

6

Your Story

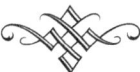

Space is provided here for you to begin to share your "vpt" story on paper.

Suggested journal topics are included in each phase of your "vpt" journey.

Take your time. Process and write in safety and peace. You are not alone!

Again, writing in your own journal book might be more appealing.

Here are the suggested emotional pain words you might especially try to use in your journaling. It will be good to try to "nail down" the exact emotions you were feeling as you journal each season of your "vpt" journey.

C.P.R.

Emotional Distress Words:

Sad	Mad	Scared
Guilty	Ashamed	Depressed
Lonely	Hurt	Hostile
Angry	Rage	Hateful
Critical	Rejected	Confused
Helpless	Submissive	Insecure
Anxious	Apathetic	Inferior
Inadequate	Miserable	Stupid
Jealous	Selfish	Frustrated
Furious	Irritated	Skeptical
Bewildered	Discouraged	Insignificant
Weak	Foolish	Embarrassed

YOUR STORY

JOURNAL EXERCISE ONE
How my journey started:

Write about circumstances surrounding your relationship with your partner. Was he your teen-age boyfriend, your college boyfriend, your husband, a one-night stand, or an affair partner? Perhaps you were married and weren't planning on this pregnancy or received an adverse diagnosis. Write as long as you wish about events leading up to the pregnancy.

_____
_____
_____
_____
_____
_____
_____
_____
_____
_____
_____
_____
_____
_____
_____
_____
_____
_____
_____
_____
_____
_____
_____

C.P.R.

The relationship continued....

Write about other events, times with your partner and the events just before the pregnancy. Write as long as you wish about events leading up to the pregnancy.

_____

_____

_____

_____

_____

_____

_____

_____

_____

_____

_____

_____

_____

_____

_____

_____

_____

_____

_____

_____

_____

_____

_____

YOUR STORY

JOURNAL EXERCISE TWO
I remember the day I found out I was pregnant…

Write about how you found out you were pregnant. Write
everything you can think of surrounding "that day." Who did
you tell? How did you feel? What were your first thoughts? What
were some other thoughts? Describe your feelings on that day
specifically.

_____

_____

_____

_____

_____

_____

_____

_____

_____

_____

_____

_____

_____

_____

_____

_____

_____

_____

_____

_____

_____

_____

_____

_____

C.P.R.

Upon finding out the news I...

Write about who you told, details of where and how you told your partner. Express all the feelings you had surrounding the news of this pregnancy. Write about feelings of responsibility you experienced. Write about reactions of those with whom you shared the news.

_____

_____

_____

_____

_____

_____

_____

_____

_____

_____

_____

_____

_____

_____

_____

_____

_____

_____

_____

_____

_____

_____

_____

YOUR STORY

JOURNAL EXERCISE THREE
Figuring out what to do…

Write about what you thought about. What did you want to do?
What did your partner want to do? What did your parents want
you to do, or were they even involved? Did you make the decision
on your own? Why? Where did you go for information? Who
suggested what? Write as many details as you can think of about
how you made your "vpt" decision.

_____

_____

_____

_____

_____

_____

_____

_____

_____

_____

_____

_____

_____

_____

_____

_____

_____

_____

_____

_____

_____

C.P.R.

The appointment was scheduled…

Write about the moments, days and weeks before the procedure.
What was going through your mind? Where was your partner?
Did you have difficulty finding help? What were you feeling?
Relief? Fear about going to your appointment?

_____

_____

_____

_____

_____

_____

_____

_____

_____

_____

_____

_____

_____

_____

_____

_____

_____

_____

_____

_____

_____

_____

_____

YOUR STORY

JOURNAL EXERCISE FOUR
The day of the appointment…

Who took you? Who went inside with you? Were you alone? What were you feeling? (Remember numb is a feeling!) What was the weather like? Where was the clinic? Write as many details as possible about "the day."

_____

_____

_____

_____

_____

_____

_____

_____

_____

_____

_____

_____

_____

_____

_____

_____

_____

_____

_____

_____

_____

_____

_____

_____

C.P.R.

JOURNAL EXERCISE FIVE
The Procedure…

This might be really hard to write about. Try to express as much
as you can about the actual event. Details might include doctors,
nurses. Try to express as much emotion as possible.

_____

_____

_____

_____

_____

_____

_____

_____

_____

_____

_____

_____

_____

_____

_____

_____

_____

_____

_____

_____

_____

YOUR STORY

JOURNAL EXERCISE SIX
Immediately afterwards…

Did you go home or where did you go? Who took you? What were you feeling, emotionally, physically? Feel free to look on your "emotional pain words list to help you identify the emotions you were feeling. What was the weather like?

_____
_____
_____
_____
_____
_____
_____
_____
_____
_____
_____
_____
_____
_____
_____
_____
_____
_____
_____
_____
_____
_____
_____
_____
_____
_____

C.P.R.

JOURNAL EXERCISE SEVEN
The days that followed…

Write about what you were feeling as the days passed after the procedure. Relief? Talk about getting back into your routine. Did you think about it? Was your partner there for you? Describe feelings, life afterwards, relationships and any other pertinent details.

_____

_____

_____

_____

_____

_____

_____

_____

_____

_____

_____

_____

_____

_____

_____

_____

_____

_____

_____

_____

_____

_____

YOUR STORY

Write about what your life was like a year later. What were you doing with your life? Who were you with? Did you think about your "vpt?" Was it "gone from your head?"

_____

_____

_____

_____

_____

_____

_____

_____

_____

_____

_____

_____

_____

_____

_____

_____

_____

_____

_____

_____

_____

_____

_____

C.P.R.

JOURNAL EXERCISE NINE
I got on with my life…

Write about life after the "vpt" decision. You can write in general about your life now or about any timeframe after your choice. Describe the person you became, what your goals were, what you were doing sometime down the road from the decision.

_____

_____

_____

_____

_____

_____

_____

_____

_____

_____

_____

_____

_____

_____

_____

_____

_____

_____

_____

_____

_____

_____

YOUR STORY

JOUNRAL EXERCISE TEN
My life today…

Write about what your life is like now…

_____

_____

_____

_____

_____

_____

_____

_____

_____

_____

_____

_____

_____

_____

_____

_____

_____

_____

_____

_____

_____

_____

_____

_____

_____

_____

_____

C.P.R.

JOURNAL EXERCISE ELEVEN
My thoughts about my "vpt"…

Write anything you like in reference to your choice decision.

_____
_____
_____
_____
_____
_____
_____
_____
_____
_____
_____
_____
_____
_____
_____
_____
_____
_____
_____
_____
_____
_____
_____
_____

YOUR STORY

JOURNAL EXERCISE TWELVE
I am giving myself permission to grieve…

Write anything you like in reference to your choice decision. You can write about your pregnancy loss. You can write about the emotions you feel when you think about your "vpt." What did you lose? What are you grieving? Let "it" all come up and out!

_____

_____

_____

_____

_____

_____

_____

_____

_____

_____

_____

_____

_____

_____

_____

_____

_____

_____

_____

_____

_____

_____

_____

_____

_____

_____

_____

C.P.R.

I am giving myself permission to grieve…

_____

_____

_____

_____

_____

_____

_____

_____

_____

_____

_____

_____

_____

_____

_____

_____

_____

_____

_____

_____

_____

_____

_____

_____

_____

_____

_____

_____

_____

_____

_____

YOUR STORY

I am giving myself permission to grieve…

_____

_____

_____

_____

_____

_____

_____

_____

_____

_____

_____

_____

_____

_____

_____

_____

_____

_____

_____

_____

_____

_____

_____

_____

_____

_____

_____

C.P.R.

I am giving myself permission to grieve…

_____
_____
_____
_____
_____
_____
_____
_____
_____
_____
_____
_____
_____
_____
_____
_____
_____
_____
_____
_____
_____
_____
_____
_____
_____
_____
_____
_____

YOUR STORY

EXERCISE THIRTEEN

Having permission to grieve and tell my story has made a
difference in my life because:

_____

_____

_____

_____

_____

_____

_____

_____

_____

_____

_____

_____

_____

_____

_____

_____

_____

_____

_____

_____

_____

_____

_____

_____

_____

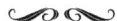

You can either choose to go through the pain of grieving your losses or you can choose to have an underlying layer of sorrow, like a low grade fever, the rest of your days.

7

Resolution

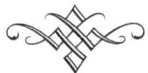

I use art therapy a lot in my practice. Any sort of creative means of expressing emotion is another very useful way to "get the emotions up and out." Remember our mission is to validate and identify emotions in a safe place. We continue to bring everything up and out. Unlocking the emotions stored in the right side of the brain helps free a person of the overwhelming grief they feel over a "vpt." For those of you who had a hard time journaling, you may have an easier time expressing yourself through this art project.

For all of you, this exercise will evoke quite a bit of emotion. That is good! Your assignment is to make two collages that will pertain to the subject of your "vpt." You will make these collages by cutting pictures, words, or phrases out of magazines. As you construct the collage let yourself feel any emotion that comes up and out. If it is anger, let the anger come. If tears stream down... that is good, good, good!

YOU CAN USE ANY SORT OF ART MATERIALS TO CONSTRUCT YOUR COLLAGE WITH. This can be a poster board material that is readily available or any other type of blank paper. It is my suggestion that you get a pretty large size piece of paper. This allows you plenty of room to "paste out" your feelings. If you are the artistic type person, you can also *draw* different aspects of what you are feeling.

❧◈❧

Collage Subjects:

<u>Collage one:</u> "On the day of my 'vpt' this is how I felt."

Try to cut out pictures that really express the emotion you felt about "that day."

Refer back to the Emotional Pain Word List if you need to identify emotions.

❧◈❧

<u>Collage two:</u> "My memorial collage."
Make a collage that memorializes your pregnancy loss.

This may even be a bit more difficult. Cut out pictures that give definition to your pregnancy. This collage could be an array of baby pictures. They could be pictures of children or hopeful pictures of scenery. Anything that describes your pregnancy loss will do. You might cut out pictures of different ages of children that would represent the different stages of life a child would go through. Again, it is important for you to feel the pain of your loss as you cut out your pictures, words and sayings.

RESOLUTION

For those of you who have had more than one "vpt" I would suggest that you make a collage for each pregnancy loss. Try to concentrate only on that particular loss as you make the collage. This is an excellent way to process each "vpt" individually. It may be that after you make the collages you can go back and do the journaling exercises for each individual "vpt."

Many of my clients take the collage they make and buy a symbol that would represent their loss to go with it. This might be a figurine or a painting or a flower arrangement. Then they make a neat memorial type presentation in their home. This brings dignity to their loss and reminds them that this event in their life was important and deserving of notice. You don't necessarily have to tell anyone else what your display represents. You will just know in your heart what it symbolizes. Publicly displaying your creation brings a sense of resolution and closure. The secret will be "out" even if it is only you who knows the true meaning. Something about symbolizing the lost pregnancy brings dignity and honor to the "vpt" experience. This is why our culture uses funerals as a way to gain closure. There is a ritual, a ceremony that draws an ending line to the loss.

C.P.R.

Collage Depicting "The Day"

RESOLUTION

Collage Depicting "The Day"

C.P.R.

MEMORIAL COLLAGE:

Paste any sort of remembrance picture or item here (ribbons, bows, dried flowers) in memory of your pregnancy loss.

RESOLUTION

MEMORIAL COLLAGE:

Paste any sort of remembrance picture or item here (ribbons, bows, dried flowers) in memory of your pregnancy loss.

C.P.R.

Memorial and Grieving Exercise

Another great way to process grief is through the use of sympathy cards. There are some really beautiful cards available. A good way to put emotion to and to make your grief a reality in your own heart is this exercise. Go to a card display. Stand in front of it and pick out the card that really speaks to the grief you are feeling about your "vpt." Bring the card home and paste it in this book or in your journaling book. Again, this is a great way to describe the sadness you feel about your "vpt."

Paste your sympathy card here:

RESOLUTION

You can't say good-bye until you've said hello.

This is your final writing project. Write a letter to your lost love. Tell your lost child hello. If you would like, give yourself permission to name your child. Express every emotion, every concern, everything and anything you would like to say. Give yourself permission to cry, shout, write and feel. Write about what you lost because of the road you chose. Write about lost hopes, lost dreams. Write about the pain. Cry the tears. Then say good-bye. And then cry some more. The tears are cleansing and healing and will bring you through to the other side, where there is closure and sunshine.

Again, it is suggested you write this letter in your actual journaling book.

Writing a Letter to My Lost Love

Dear _____,

Good-bye_____

C.P.R.

I would be amiss if I weren't vulnerable enough to share with you, the readers, my own letter to my daughter, Jesse Lynn. It is short but what I needed to say at the time to reach a place of resolution.

Dear Jesse Lynn,

This letter is to let you know how much I love you. Though I never met you, I know I love you. I am feeling so many feelings about your loss. I was so young and scared and I didn't think the "time was right" for you. I was at a place in my life where I thought no one cared. I took what I thought would be the best path for everyone involved.

Just know that you are missed; there will always be a hole in my heart for you. Your life was a pebble that dropped in the water. The ripples go forth and rock my heart with sadness. Each wave passes through and I know you were an important person in our family and you will always be missed.

I think of what your life could have been and I am so sad. I see you as an energetic toddler with curly blonde hair. I see you going to school that first day. I see you playing soccer, having fun with friends, going on that first date, the prom, and even as a young adult finishing college. You wear your bride's dress elegantly.

I am writing this letter to acknowledge you and then to tell you good-bye. I realize I needed to tell you hello first, though. Just know that I am finally letting myself cry. It is so hard to go to this deep place of pain in my heart, but I know going through the pain is what I need to do.

For now, I say "hello" to you. And after I cry, I will once again say "good-bye." I hope you know I loved you and that you were missed.

Love from your Mom,

Summary

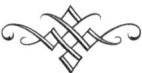

Community and Belonging

Voluntary pregnancy termination can create a deep sense of loss for women. Unfortunately, the ideological and political positions of the "A-word" in and of itself puts the women who make a "vpt" choice in a place of disenfranchisement.

Those who sanction the legalities of the procedure don't necessarily understand the aftermath of grief that can follow a decision.

Conversely, those who don't believe in choice usually concentrate on the legal and moral aspects of choice. Somewhere in-between, women walk alone in their effort to resolve the grief surrounding their loss. The controversy, the rhetoric, the political hees and haws put the very person both sides are trying to help in a difficult position.

Disenfranchised grief falls in the category of Type-A trauma. Type-A trauma isn't necessarily trauma in the grand sense of the word. In this case, the word trauma refers to the Greek metaphor meaning "wound." Any type of pain that involves a "lack of" qualifies as a Type-A trauma. A lack of recognition for the eventual grief a "vpt" brings is what causes women who make the choice have confusion and difficulty processing the underlying sadness that might appear years later after their decision.

Type-A trauma happens within the confines of a sense of "aloneness." Conversely, type-A trauma can best be resolved within a sense of community. It is for this reason, after you have worked through this grief process, it will be advisable by this therapist/author that you go further down the road by connecting with others who are in your same place.

After you have worked through a lot of grief concerning your "vpt" you may want to consider getting involved in a support group. Support groups are a proven method for helping reach closure in grief situations. I hope this book has served its purpose in getting the top layer of grief off. Perhaps now you are motivated to take your journey one step further. Getting involved in a group setting will further dispel the disenfranchisement you might feel concerning your "vpt."

It was the person who first cried with me that told me about a support group in my area. (I had no clue they existed!). The first meeting I parked down the street. I walked up the alley and went in the back door. How ironic! Once in the room, though, what a freeing experience! For the first time in my life I talked with others who felt like I did. All those years I thought I was alone!

If you think you are ready to be involved in a support group, please know non-judgmental groups are available. You can go to my Web site, www.missingpieces.org and choose "contact us." Check the "request for a referral to a support group in your area" button. I will do my best to find safe, nonjudgmental support for you.

SUMMARY

WHAT ABOUT PROFESSIONAL THERAPY?

Missing Pieces.Org is dedicated to training and informing professional therapists about the issue of grief after abortion. You might consider having a professional walk with you through the grief process. I have developed a treatment plan professionals can use to help their clients take this journey. You can take your "CPR" self-help book to your therapist and inform them of the companion book developed especially for professionals to use with their clients.

∽∂∽

CHOICE PROCESSING AND RESOLUTION THERAPY

TREATMENT PLAN FOR PROFESSIONALS:
Choice Processing and Resolution Therapy is an excellent resource your professional therapist can use to help them understand the disenfranchisement of grief after "vpt."

Your therapist can go to www.amazon.com and download the kindle version of this resource. Simply type in "Choice Processing and Resolution Therapy Trudy Johnson" in the book search to order from amazon.

FORMS FOR PROFESSIONALS:
In addition, your therapist can go to www.missingpieces.org/professionals to download forms they can use with you as you process "vpt" grief together.

C.P.R.

CONTACT MISSING PIECES:

Your therapist can go the "Contact Us" form on the www.missingpieces.org website and submit questions or request a hard copy of the treatment plan.

A PERSONAL WORD FROM TRUDY

I can't stress enough that you are not alone in your journey to process your "vpt" grief. Here are two parting words of advice I have for you:

GET BACK TO YOUR FAITH: If you have felt disconnected in your faith because you have experienced guilt, shame or condemnation, I would encourage you to return to your roots. I hope this book has helped you work past your sense of shame and guilt. These are difficult times and we all need a compass and an anchor. Return to your faith with a new sense of freedom from shame. Feeling condemned does none of us any good, so don't!

FEEL FREE TO CONTACT ME with "your story" or any comments you have about *"C.P.R."* I would love to hear what you have to say. The email address is missingpiecesorg@gmail.com. I could not feel more honored than to have been a small part of your personal journey to resolution.

❦

"May peace and grace be with you in full measure."
Your "vpt sister," Trudy

❦

ABOUT THE AUTHOR

Trudy M. Johnson, M.A., L.M.F.T.,C.S.P.M.L., is a licensed Marriage and Family Therapist in the state of Colorado. She is in private practice working with persons suffering from depression, effects of abuse and trauma and emotional regulation. She offers Brief Intensive Therapy for women and in the heart of the Rocky Mountains of Colorado. For more information go to www.anesisretreats.com.

She also conducts week-long counseling sabbaticals at a Christian retreat center for trauma related to sexual abuse or abortion grief. For more information visit www.anesisretreats.com.

C.P.R.

Tell a friend or loved one about this book as a resource to help them process grief they may be feeling after their "vpt."

RESOURCES:

www.sadafterabortion.com

www.missingpieces.org
Resources for professional therapists and individuals

https://www.facebook.com/dealingwithgriefafterabortion
Private message Trudy or read encouraging thoughts on abortion grief here.

http://www.yourtango.com/experts/trudyjohnson
Read Trudy's blogs about abortion grief

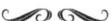

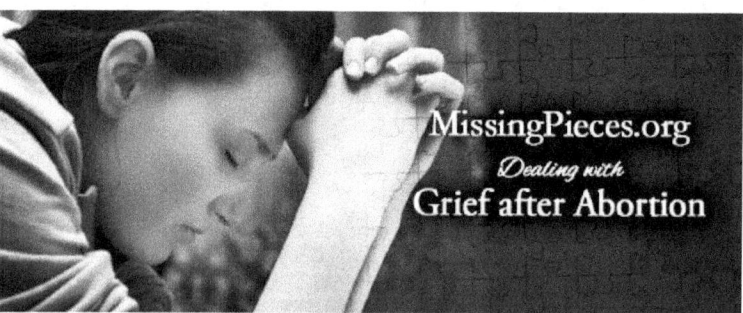

Go to www.missingpieces.org and choose the "Contact Us" tab to request resources, get a referral for a support group or sign up for our quarterly newsletter.

Upcoming Resources:

"Nunca Tienes Que Sentirte Solitaria Por Este Camino"

The Spanish version of CPR ~ Choice Processing and Resolution is available Spring 2014. We are excited to offer this resource to Spanish-speaking women world-wide. Check www.amazon.com for the Kindle version.

"C.P.R." for Men

Choice processing and resolution surrounding the issue of voluntary pregnancy termination with a new understanding and resolution tips for men involved in a "vpt" decision.

Publish Date: Spring 2015

C.P.R.

TO CONTACT TRUDY

Struggling?

Feel free to email Trudy with your thoughts,
comments and "vpt" struggles

missingpiecesorg@gmail.com

NOTES: